NATURAL BIRTH

Acknowledgements

Acknowledgment is gratefully made to the following publications in which selections from this book appear: *Chrysalis, Extended Outlooks, The Iowa Review* and *Sinister Wisdom*.

I would like to thank the MacDowell Colony for its support, the New Jersey State Council on the Arts for a grant which helped me complete some of these poems, and the many women whose encouragement, criticism and suggestions kept me going. In particular, I would like to thank those who were the first to see this manuscript and to believe in its possibilities: Bruce Derricotte, Vera Raynor, Jan Kweit, Marilyn Hacker and Sharon Olds.

NATURAL BIRTH

Poems
by
Toi Derricotte

 The Crossing Press / Trumansburg, New York 14886

The Crossing Press Feminist Series

Toi Derricotte is the author of a collection of poetry,
The Empress of the Death House (Lotus Press, 1978).

Copyright © 1983 by Toi Derricotte

Book and cover design by Mary A. Scott

Photograph of Toi Derricotte by Nat Clymer, *Somerset Messenger Gazette*

Typesetting by Martha J. Waters

Library of Congress Cataloging in Publication Data

Derricotte, Toi, 1941-
    Natural birth.

    (Crossing Press feminist series)
    1. Childbirth--Poetry. I. Title. II. Series.
PS3554.E73N3 1983 811'.54   83-2071
ISBN 0-89594-102-3
ISBN 0-89594-101-5 (pbk.)

For my son, Tony

CONTENTS

please, god, make it easy,
i said it would be easy.
i don't want a shot. i
want it to be beautiful
like it's supposed to be . . .

NATURAL BIRTH

In my seventh month, I traveled to a maternity home in
another city. When I arrived, there was no room until
December. I was placed with the Reynolds family until
space was available.

November

nun meets me at the station. first month with carol and
dick reynolds. *set the table. clean the kitchen. vacuum.*
thank god she didn't ask me to take care of the children.

i dry dishes in the afternoon. watch her can apples from
the backyard, put them in the cellar dark to save for winter.

why is everything so quiet? why does the man come home
from school every day at 3:30 and read the paper? why a
different casserole on the table every night and everyone
eats one portion and one portion only? why is there always
enough, but never too much . . .

try to understand this quiet, busy woman. is she content?
what are her reasons to can, to cook, to have three children
and a pregnant girl in her house? try to be close, lie
next to their quiet ticking bedroom, and hear no sound,

night after night, except soft conversation. in the morning,
before light, i hear the baby's first cry. i picture her
in there with her bra unhooked and her heavy white breast
like cream on the cheek of that baby.

inside i wonder what she thinks, feels, who she is. and
every night it gets dark earlier, stays dark later. i don't
want to wake up smiling at cereal. dark overshadows snow,
and a fear comes into my cold heart: *i am alone.*

one afternoon, drying dishes, her cutting apples by the
sink, i ask her about college. i picture her so easily
in penny loafers, peck and peck collar, socks, and a plaid
skirt on her skinny still unchilded body. here she is today
with hips and breasts, a woman thirty who had taught school—
she must have some thoughts, some arguments and passions
hidden in this kitchen.

finally, she tells me her favorite book is <u>the stranger</u>.
we go and find it on the living room shelf. i wonder,
though she never says, what she understands about
being a stranger . . .

i meet her mother—all the same—they treat me all
the same: human. i am accepted, never question who
i am or why. never make me feel unwanted or afraid.
but always human love and never passion, never clutching
need, lopsided devouring want, never, not one minute,
extending those boundaries to enclose me . . .

                                        oh soul,

                                                  i feel
cold and unused to such space as breath and eternity
around me . . .
                    so much room in silence . . .

how will <u>my</u> house ever run on silence, when in me there
is such noise, such hatred for peeling apples, canning,
and waking to feed baby, and alarm clocks in the soul, and
in the skin of baby, in the rind of oranges, apples, peels
in the garbage, and paper saved because it is cheaper to
save and wrap and wash and use everything again. and clean,
no screaming in that house, no tears, one helping at dinner,
and no lovemaking noises like broken squeaky beds. where is
that part i cannot touch no matter where or how i turn,
that part that wants to cry: *SISTER,* and make us touch . . .

she is kind. though i never understand such kindness.
cannot understand the inner heart of how and why she
loves: *i am the stranger.*

somewhere in the back of my mind, they are either fools
or the holy family, the way we all should be if we lived
in a perfect world and didn't have to strive to be loved,
but went about our quiet business, never raising our voices
above the rest, never questioning if we are loved, or
whether what we do is what we want to do, or worth it . . .

and if they are fools who don't have hearts or brains
or cords in their necks to speak, then why have they
asked for me? why am i in their house? why are they
doing this?

one night in my round black coat and leotards, i dress
up warm against the constellations, go down the snowy
block alone in time. i am only going to the drugstore,
but for some reason, the way i feel, pregnantly beautiful
walking into the bright fluorescent drugstore, it is
the most vivid night in my mind in the whole darkening
november . . .

In my ninth month, I entered a maternity ward set up for
the care of unwed girls and women in Holy Cross Hospital.

Holy Cross Hospital

couldn't stand to see these new young faces, these
children swollen as myself. my roommate, snotty,
bragging about how she didn't give a damn about the
kid and was going back to her boyfriend and be a
cheerleader in high school. *could we ever "go back"?*
would our bodies be the same? could we hide among the
childless? she always reminded me of a lady at the bridge
club in her mother's shoes, playing her mother's hand.

i tried to get along, be silent, stay in my own corner.
i only had a month to go—too short to get to know them.
but being drawn to the room down the hall, the t.v. room
where, at night, we sat in our cuddly cotton robes and
fleece-lined slippers—like college freshmen, joking
about the nuns and laughing about due dates: jailbirds
waiting to be sprung . . .

one girl, taller and older, twenty-six or twenty-seven, kept
to herself, talked with a funny accent. the pain on her face
seemed worse than ours . . .

and a lovely, gentle girl with flat small bones. the
great round hump seemed to carry her around! she never
said an unkind word to anyone, went to church every morning
with her rosary and prayed each night alone in her room.

she was seventeen, diabetic, fearful that she or the baby
or both would die in childbirth. she wanted the baby, yet
knew that to keep it would be wrong. but what if the child
did live? what if she gave it up and could never have another?

i couldn't believe the fear, the knowledge she had of
death walking with her. i never felt stronger, eating
right, doing my exercises. i was holding on to the core,
the center of strength; death seemed remote, i could not
imagine it walking in our midst, death in the midst of
all that blooming. she seemed sincere, but maybe she
was lying . . .

she went down two weeks late. induced. she had decided
to keep the baby. the night i went down, she had just
gone into labor so the girls had two of us to cheer about.
the next morning when i awoke, i went to see her. she
smiled from her hospital bed with tubes in her arms. it
had been a boy. her baby was dead in the womb for two
weeks. i remembered she had complained *no kicking*. we
had reassured her everything was fine.

meanwhile i worked in the laundry, folded the hospital
fresh sheets flat three hours a day. but never alone.
stepping off the elevator, going up, feeling something,
a spark catch. i would put my hand there and smile with
such a luminous smile, the whole world must be happy.

or out with those crazy girls, those teenagers, laughing,
on a christmas shopping spree, free (the only day they
let us out in two months) feet wet and cold from snow.

i felt pretty, body wide and still in black beatnik
leotards, washed out at night. my shapely legs and
young body like iron.

i ate well, wanted lamaze (painless childbirth)—i
didn't need a husband or a trained doctor—i'd do it
myself, book propped open on the floor, puffing and
counting while all the sixteen-year-old unwed children
smiled like i was crazy.

one day i got a letter from my cousin, said:

> *don't give your baby up—*
> *you'll never be complete again*
> *you'll always worry where and how it is*

she knew! the people in my family knew! nobody died
of grief and shame!

i <u>would</u> keep the child. i was sturdy. would be a better
mother than my mother. i would still be a doctor,
study, finish school at night. when the time came, i
would not hurt like all those women who screamed and
took drugs. I would squat down and deliver just like the
peasants in the field, shift my baby to my back, and
continue . . .

when my water broke, when i saw that stain of pink blood
on the toilet paper and felt the first thing i could not
feel, had no control of, dripping down my leg, i heard
them singing mitch miller xmas songs and came from the
bathroom in my own pink song—down the long hall, down
the long moment when no one knew but me. it was time.

all the girls were cheering when i went downstairs. i was
the one who told them to be tough, to stop believing
in their mother's pain, that poison. our minds were
like telescopes looking through fear. it wouldn't hurt
like we'd been told. birth was beautiful if we believed
that it was beautiful and right and good!

—maternity—i had never seen inside those doors.
all night i pictured the girls up there, at first hanging
out of the windows, trying to get a glimpse of me . . .
when the pain was worst, i thought of their sleeping faces,
like the shining faces of children in the nursery. i held
onto that image of innocence like one light in the darkness.

pain is as common as flies. if you don't see it
walking on your lip, if you can't breathe it,
don't feel it for yourself, you walk in darkness.
not knowing the price of common sunshine, common
air, the common footstep on the earth. one
moment of life must be paid for, and no one
walking in the darkness without eyes can see.

the child is cut off from the mother, cut off
from the blinding pain the mother sleeps
and wakes up in forever, balancing the asshole
of the universe, the abyss of god's brain, inside
that light in her forehead.

she is bright. so bright that everything must
turn and face her like the sun. every clock
in life must stop to let her pass. slowly,
like the regal death procession of the king.

Maternity

when they checked me in, i was thinking: *this is going to be
a snap!* but at the same time, everything looked so different!
this was another world, ordered and white. the night moved
by on wheels.

suddenly the newness of the bed, the room, the quiet,
the hospital gown they put me in, the sheets rolled up
hard and starched and white and everything white except the
clock on the wall in red and black and the nurse's back as
she moved out of the room without speaking, everything
conspired to make me feel afraid.

how long, how much will i suffer?

the night looked in from bottomless windows.

10:29

going to the bathroom. worse than cramps. can't stop
going to the bathroom. shaking my head over the toilet.
just sit. sit on the toilet. don't move. just shake
your head. try to go so hard. maybe it will go away.
just try. press real hard. *it hurts   i can't help it   oh
it hurts so bad!*

lie on the bed and can't breathe right. go to sleep and
wake up in the middle of a wave, too late . . .

what time is it, i can't keep track of time . . .

fall asleep. two minutes. can't stand the pain. have
to go to the bathroom. feels so ugly pressing down there,
shame, shame! have to go to the bathroom all the time.
shake my head. can't believe it hurts like this and
getting worse.

lie back in bed, just breathe. just relax. watch the
clock. one minute goes so slow. seems like 10:29, the
clock is stuck there, stuck on pain . . .

nurse comes in, asks me if i want a shot. *no i don't want a shot. i want this to be easy. please god make it easy, i said it would be easy. no i don't want a shot don't want to give up yet, i want it to be beautiful like it's supposed to be if i just breathe right, can't give up they want me to give up i won't give up* (the minutes stuck around the clock), *please nobody see me* (the nurse says the social worker wants to see me . . . and the social worker is pregnant!) *god don't let her see. i told her to have lamaze like me told her it was easy and not to be afraid. don't let her see how hard don't let her be afraid like i am now. never again, never have a baby, never believe that this is beautiful or right or good i'm rolling in the dark the clock is stuck the big black clock is stuck all night. inside i'm quiet outside i roll and can't stop it getting worse, can't stop it's getting worse—it can't get worse! how could a body hold such pain? how could such pain be here and how and what did i do? i want to scream i can't. my mouth is stopped my mouth is dry— so dry god let me out of this hell i did my exercises loved my baby did everything i could, you promised if i was good you promised if i was clean and pure and beautiful, if i was humble like a child and loved them all the little children* (so far to the bathroom, so cold in the night loving my baby, so far, so cold, so long) *and no one to come and save me from this pain i cannot stop oh god no one to save me . . . .*

i watch the clock. 10:29. wait, desperate to see time go. it all depends on time. everything depends on those black lines on the clock. the second hand goes round. i want to push it, pray it into place.

between each second are millions of seconds that must
be touched and passed. the clock goes no where. or
else i look again, and it has gone back.

time is going nowhere   only me inside of time is getting
deeper   getting lost   can't skate across the hours forgetting
memory of pain   no where to hide   each moment is a desert
i must cross   can't find the sides of anything   everything
expanding growing wider larger   only me inside of time is
growing smaller   disappearing in a wider hole of nothing
i have never been alive before, never want to be alive again . . .

doctor comes in, wrenches his hand, a hammer up my cunt.
wants to feel the head, wants to feel the damn thing's
head, wants to see how far i am. and i roll and moan
and beg him not to see, but he keeps "seeing." (no
pain like this ever.) and i am thinking, *this is the one*
who told me i would hurt. FORGET ALL THAT SILLY
BREATHING STUFF. YOU'LL TAKE A SHOT LIKE THE
REST WHEN THE TIME COMES. now, every time he
sticks that wooden board up me, jams that stake inside my
bleeding heart, i know, this is one who likes to give me pain.

this is static. no stop between. how can they know the
mountain of pain in me? how can every woman suffer so?
how can every man and woman walking on legs, the thousands
you see each day, how can each have had a mother like me?
how can life contain it? how can any woman know and let
this happen? one pain like this should be enough to save
the world forever.

the nurse says she'll give me a shot. still wants to
give me a shot. *but i don't want a shot. i've tried so hard
all night to stay awake and fight and breathe, and now it's
8:00 and might go on like this forever   i want to be awake
and see my baby, want to see him crown, the head immense
as sun and bright with blood crack over the bowl of earth   i
want to feel the womb of god close over me, and want to,
more than anything, feel joy and love and welcome him   god
help this man be born into this world   help   his mother wants
to share this moment with his beauty   wants to hold on to
the pain a second more and feel him crown inside me   majesty
and might   no more than being humble will allow a broken
woman, let me be awake and push him into light . . .*

*it's light outside   it's light   i can see it in the mirror
day is coming   night is passing   i am so far in myself
i can't see out   can't say no to anything floating on my
pain . . .*

doctor comes in to feel the head. keeps coming in,
making me hurt, sticking his whole hand up my asshole.
and it hurts like sticking a wooden ax handle up my cunt
and grinding it inside me, hot cigars burning ax handles
and i can't move i'm in such pain, can't move away from
him raping me each time sticking his whole gloved hand
up my wounded cunt.

my heart is open. my whole body is open and cannot say
no. my mouth, each mouth inside me is open and bleeding.
each heart is like the moon without a middle, a white
hole in the sky so wide the sun has gone through.

he must be happy to make me feel such pain. he must be
happy because he is a man and in control of me and i
cannot move away from him while he takes me on this bed
of pain and he tells me it is for my own good when i
tell him how i hurt, he tells me it is almost over, but
the clock is stuck on pain, stuck on forever, and i know
that he is lying.

he wants me to roll and beg like a dog, *please doctor
please don't hurt me any more   do anything   do anything you
say   but help me   help me not to feel such pain*   but i don't
beg him. i don't beg him because i hate him. i keep
my pain locked up inside. he'll never know how much
he hurts, i'll never let him know.

my heart is frozen like a calf. on ice. my heart is
empty meat. my heart, my love is frozen. i will never
love again.

up there. the girls are in the dark. behind
dark panes of glass. i cannot look in, but
i can see their faces. they are happy for me.
they have gone to sleep with smiles on their
faces. they are happy because i have
gone down.

but i am so alone.

tonight all windows are grey and shuttered
like paper. all rooms are closed to me tonight
except this room, awash with brightness.

far away, across the courtyard, up through
darkness, like the dark around a ship without
a thought of land, is light, another light, the
light of girls' dreams.

how i wish that one would light a candle,
all night a candle of consciousness lit
outside my pain. but i am far away, lost to
the sight of land, and they are quiet, like
children in the nursery.

let them sleep tonight, ignorant of where i
stand (their knowledge cannot help). but how
will i ever look beauty in the face again,
once blinded by this light?

Transition

the meat rolls up and moans on the damp table.
my body is a piece of cotton over another
woman's body. some other woman, all muscle and nerve, is
tearing apart and opening under me.

i move with her like skin, not able to do anything else,
i am just watching her, not able to believe what her
body can do, what it <u>will</u> do, to get this thing accomplished.

this muscle of a lady, this crazy ocean in my teacup.
she moves the pillars of the sky. i am stretched into
fragments, tissue paper thin. the light shines through
to her goatness, her blood-thick heart that thuds like
one drum in the universe emptying its stars.

she is
that heart
larger
than my life

stuffed
in
me
like sausage
black sky
bird
pecking
at the bloody
ligament

trying
to get
in, get
out
i am

holding out with
everything i
have
holding out
the evil thing

when i see there is
no answer
to the screamed
word
GOD
nothing i can do,
no use,

i have to let her in,
open the door,
put down the mat
welcome her
as if she
might be the
called for death,
the final
abstraction.

she comes
like a tunnel
fast
coming into
blackness
with my headlights
off

   you can push . . .

i hung there. still hurting, not knowing what to do.
if you push too early, it hurts more. i called the
doctor back again. *are you sure i can push? are you sure?*

i couldn't believe that pain was over, that the punish-
ment was enough, that the wave, the huge blue mind i
was living inside, was receding. i had forgotten there
ever was a life without pain, a moment when pain wasn't
absolute as air.

why weren't the nurses and doctors rushing toward me?
why weren't they wrapping me in white? white for respect,
white for triumph, white for the white light i was being
accepted into after death? why was it so simple as saying
you can push? why were they walking away from me into
other rooms as if this were not the end the beginning of
something which the world should watch?

i felt something pulling me inside, a soft call, but i
could feel her power. something inside me i could go
with, wide and deep and wonderful. the more i gave
to her, the more she answered me. i held this conversation
in myself like a love that never stops. i pushed toward
her, she came toward me, gently, softly, sucking like a
wave. i pushed deeper and she swelled wider, darker when
she saw i wasn't afraid. then i saw the darker glory
of her under me.

why wasn't the room bursting with lilies? why was
everything the same with them moving so slowly as if
they were drugged? why were they acting the same when,
suddenly, everything had changed?

we were through with pain, would never suffer in our
lives again. put pain down like a rag, unzipper skin,
step out of our dead bodies, and leave them on the
floor. glorious spirits were rising, blanched with
light, like thirsty women shining with their thirst.

i felt myself rise up with all the dead, climb out of
the tomb like christ, holy and wise, transfigured with
the knowledge of the tomb inside my brain, holding the
gold key to the dark stamped inside my genes, never to
be forgotten . . .

it was time. it was really time. this baby would be
born. it would really happen. this wasn't just a
trick to leave me in hell forever. like all the other
babies, babies of women lined up in rooms along the halls,
semi-conscious, moaning, breathing, alone with or without
husbands, there was a natural end to it that i was going
to live to see! soon i would believe in something larger
than pain, a purpose and an end. i had lived through to
another mind, a total revolution of the stars, and had
come out on the other side!

one can only imagine the shifting of the universe, the
layers of shale and rock and sky torturing against each
other, the tension, the sudden letting go. the pivot of
one woman stuck in the socket, flesh and bones giving
way, the v-groin locked, vise thigh, and the sudden
release when everything comes to rest on new pillars.

where is the woman who left home one night at 10 p.m.
while everyone was watching the mitch miller xmas show?
lost to you, to herself, to everyone

they finished watching the news, went to sleep,
dreamed, woke up, pissed, brushed their teeth, ate
corn flakes, combed their hair, and on the way out
of the door, they got a phone call . . .

while they slept the whole universe had changed.

Delivery

i was in the delivery room. PUT YOUR
FEET UP IN THE STIRRUPS. i put them up, obedient
still humbled, though the spirit was growing larger
in me, that black woman was in my throat, her thin
song, high pitched like a lark, and all the muscles
were starting to constrict around her.
i tried to push just a little. it
didn't hurt. i tried a little more.

ROLL UP, guzzo said. he wanted to give me
a spinal. NO. I DON'T WANT A SPINAL. (same
doctor as ax handle up my butt, same as shaft
of split wood, doctor spike, driving the
head home where my soft animal cowed and prayed and
cried for his mother.)

or was the baby
part of this
whole damn
conspiracy,
in on it with
guzzo,
the two of them
wanting to shoot
the wood
up me for
nothing,

for playing
music to him
in the dark
for singing
to my round
clasped
belly
for filling
up with
pizza on a cold
night, dough
warm.

maybe
he
wanted
out,
was saying
give her
a needle
and let me/the hell/
out of here
who cares
what she
wants
put her
to sleep.

                              (my baby
                              pushing off
                              with his black
                              feet
                              from the dark
                              shore, heading
                              out, not
                              knowing
                              which way and trusting,
                              oarless and eyeless, so
                              hopeless
                              it didn't matter.)

no. not
my baby.
this
loved
thing
in/ and of
myself

so i balled up
and let him
try to
stick it in.
                maybe
something was
wrong

     ROLL UP
he said
     ROLL UP
but i don't want it
     ROLL UP ROLL UP
but it doesn't hurt

we all stood,
nurses, round the white
light
hands
hanging
empty at our sides
     ROLL UP IN A BALL
all of us not
knowing
how
or if
in such a world without
false promises
we could say
anything
but, *yes,*
yes.
come take it
and be quick.

i put my belly in my hand
gave him that
thin side
of my back
the bones
intruding on the air
in little knobs
in joints
he might
crack
down my spine
his knuckles
rap
each twisted
symmetry
put me on
the rack,
each
nerve
bright
and stretched
like canvas.

he couldn't get it in!
three times, he tried
ROLL UP, he cried, ROLL UP
three times
he couldn't get it in!

dr. y (the head obstetrician)
came in

*"what are you
doing, guzzo,
i thought she
wanted
natural . . .*

(to me) *do
you want
a shot . . . no? well,*

*PUT YOUR LEGS UP,
GIRL, AND
PUSH!"*

and suddenly, the light
went out
the nurses
laughed
and nothing
mattered
in this 10
a.m. sun
shiny morning
we were well
the nurses and the
doctors cheering
that girl

combing hair
all in one
direction
shining
bright as water.

     i
grew deep
in me
like fist and i
grew deep
in me
like death
     and i
grew deep
in me
like hiding in the sea and
i was
over me
like
sun and i
was under
me
like sky and i
could look
into myself
like one
dark eye.

        i was her
and she was me
and we were
scattered round
like light
        nurses
        doctors
cheering

                such waves

my face
contorted,
never
wore
such mask, so
rigid
and so dark
        so
bright, un-
compromising
brave
no turning
back/no
no's.

i was so
beautiful. i
could look
up in the
light and
see my huge-
ness,
arc,
electric,
heavy, fleshy, living
light.

no wonder they
praised me,
a gesture
one makes
helpless and
urgent, praising
what goes on
without our praise.

when there
was nowhere
i could go, when i
was so deep
in myself
so large
i had to

let it out
they said
      drop back. i

dropped back
on the table
panting,
they moved
the head, swiveled
it correctly

      but i

         i

was
loosing
her. something
    a head
coming through
the door.
NAME PLEASE/
PLEASE / NAME / whose

head / i
don't know / some /
      disconnection

        NAME PLEASE /

and i
am not ready:

the sudden visibility—
his body,
his curly wet hair,
his arms
abandoned in that air,
an arching, squiggling thing,
his skin must be
so cold,
but there is nothing
i can do
to warm him,
his body clutches
in a wretched
spineless way.

they expect me
to sing
joy   joy
a son is born,
child is given.
tongue
curled in my head
tears, cheeks
stringy with
damp hair.

this lump
of flesh,
lump of steamy
viscera.

who

is this
child

who

is his father

a child
never having
been seen
before,
without
credentials
credit cards without
employee
reference or
high school grades or
anything
to make him
human make
him mine but
skein of
pain to
chop off
at the navel.

while they could
they held him down and
chopped him, held him up
my little fish, my blueness
swallowed in the air
turned pink
and wailed.

no more. enough.
i lay back, speechless, looking
for something

to say to myself.

after you have
touched the brain,
that squirmy
lust of maggots,
after you have
pumped the heart,
that thief,
that comic, you
throw her in the trash.

and the little one
in a case
of glass . . .

        he is not i
        i am not him
        he is not i

. . . the stranger . . .

blue
air
protects us from each other.

here.
here is the note he brings.
it says, *"mother."*

but i do not even know
this man.

POSTPARTUM

The Presentation

they wheeled her out of the delivery room on a silver cart,
a piece of limp meat without a soul. when she woke the
day was fine crystal filaments shaking itself around
her.

she waited for something wrapped like a package, something
that knew its name better than she knew it; a thing she
had to discover, to unwrap and count, slowly, parting the
visible.

under her gown, the body of a stranger fed itself, sucked
moisture into her breasts, collapsed her womb like dried
eggplant.

a new muscle shaped her, clamped itself over her being.
whatever was left, hung limp: a dumb creature, numbly
attending.

The Visiting Hour

he came in his seedy brown jacket smelling of paint. all
thumbs, a man stumbling over his own muscles, unable to
hold some part of himself and rock it, gently. she gave
up, seeing him come in the door, wanting to show him her
flat belly just an hour before, looking at her own corpse
in the mirror. she lay there reduced, neither virgin nor mother.

it had been decided. the winter was too cold in the garage.
they would live with her mother. the old bedroom was
already prepared, cleaned, the door opened. the solitary
twin bed remained; he would sleep on the porch.

she looked at him and tried to feel her way into the body
of a woman, a thing which was to be taken care of, held
safely in his arms . . .

she lay there, trying to hold on to what she had, knowing
she had to let it go.

Leaving

she never went back to the ward for the girls, except
during the day when they were all in the laundry
room, working. everything seemed anticlimactic; the
tall thin one she passed in the hall spoke as if
she hardly knew her.

where did those girls go after the births of their
babies? what wind blew them away like ashes? those
she loved well, without question; those she was
taught not to believe in, the whore, where did they
go when they were flat and empty, when they fit back
into their old clothes?

like shamed nuns, they left the dormitory, silent.
their clothes were delivered in a paper sack, and
they dressed hurriedly in the dark. the papers had
been signed. most had asked to be blindfolded.

downstairs, in the laundry, creatures like giant
insects continued to hum and move their metal arms.
the ones that were left fed them like robots.

IN
KNOWLEDGE
OF
YOUNG
BOYS

In Knowledge
of Young Boys

i knew you before you had a mother,
when you were newtlike, swimming,
a horrible brain in water.
i knew you when your connections
belonged only to yourself,
when you had no history
to hook on to,
barnacle,
when you had no sustenance of metal
when you had no boat to travel
when you stayed in the same
place, treading the question;
i knew you when you were all
eyes and a cocktail,
blank as the sky of a mind,
a root, neither ground nor placental;
not yet
red with the cut nor astonished
by pain, one terrible eye
open in the center of your head
to night, turning, and the stars
blinked like a cat. we swam
in the last trickle of champagne
before we knew breastmilk—we
shared the night of the closet,

the parasitic
closing on our thumbprint,
we were smudged in a yellow book.

son, we were oak without
mouth, uncut, we were
brave before memory.

Natural Birth, Poems by Toi Derricotte, is part of The Crossing Press Feminist Series. Other titles in this Series include:

Feminist Calendars

Folly, A Novel by Maureen Brady

Learning Our Way: Essays in Feminist Education, edited by Charlotte Bunch and Sandra Pollack

Lesbian Images, Literary Commentary by Jane Rule

Mother, Sister, Daughter, Lover, Stories by Jan Clausen

Motherwit: A Feminist Guide to Psychic Development by Diane Mariechild

Movement, A Novel by Valerie Miner

The Notebooks of Leni Clare and Other Short Stories by Sandy Boucher

The Politics of Reality: Essays in Feminist Theory by Marilyn Frye

The Queen of Wands, Poetry by Judy Grahn

True to Life Adventure Stories, Volumes I and II, edited by Judy Grahn